Lupus Diet Solutions

Proven Strategies to Heal Your Body with Anti-Inflammatory Recipes for Symptom Relief.

Angela. O.

© 2024 Angela O. All rights reserved.

No part of this book may be reproduced, distributed, or transmitted in any form or by any means, including photocopying, recording, or other electronic or mechanical methods, without the prior written permission of the author, except in the case of brief quotations embodied in critical reviews and certain other noncommercial uses permitted by copyright law.

<u>**Angela. O.**</u>

Introduction

Understanding Lupus: What You Should Know

Lupus is a chronic autoimmune illness that affects millions of individuals worldwide. Its unpredictable nature makes it a particularly difficult condition to manage because it can affect many different systems in the body, including the skin, joints, and internal organs. The term "lupus" refers to numerous different types of the disease, the most prevalent being systemic lupus erythematosus (SLE), which can cause a variety of symptoms ranging from moderate to life-threatening.

For many people, their lupus journey begins with a slew of inexplicable symptoms, including exhaustion, joint pain, and skin rashes. These symptoms frequently change, resulting in periods of remission and flare-ups. Lupus is thought to be caused by a combination of genetic, environmental, and hormonal factors, however the exact origin is unknown.

Understanding lupus entails not only recognizing the symptoms, but also appreciating the broader impact illness can have on a person's quality of life. The emotional toll can be severe, with many people experiencing anxiety and sadness as a result of the disease's chronicity and unpredictability.

Finding appropriate management options is critical for lupus patients. This is when dietary options come into play. According to research, nutrition has a substantial impact on inflammation and immunological function, both of which are important in treating lupus symptoms.

Diet is important for managing lupus symptoms.

The foods we eat can either benefit or harm our health, especially when it comes to managing autoimmune diseases such as Lupus. While there is no "cure" for lupus, following an anti-inflammatory diet can help alleviate symptoms and improve overall health.

According to studies, certain foods might promote inflammation in the body, resulting in greater lupus symptoms. In contrast, a diet high in whole, nutrient-dense foods can help reduce inflammation and strengthen the immune system. This idea emphasizes the significance of being deliberate about food choices.

Anti-inflammatory foods provide elements that assist reduce inflammation. These foods include fresh fruits and vegetables, entire grains, healthy fats, and lean proteins. Fatty fish high in omega-3 fatty acids, such salmon and mackerel, have been demonstrated to help reduce inflammation.

Consuming a range of colored fruits and vegetables can also deliver antioxidants, which fight oxidative stress and promote cellular health.

Identifying Trigger Foods: While some foods can promote healing, others can cause flare-ups. Processed foods high in sugar, trans fats, and refined carbohydrates are common culprits, and they can lead to increased inflammation and negatively impact overall health. It's also important to be aware of food sensitivities, such as gluten or dairy, which can vary from person to person.

Probiotic-rich foods, such as yogurt and sauerkraut, can help manage lupus by supporting a healthy gut microbiome. Proper hydration is essential for overall health and can help reduce lupus symptoms. Gut health is also important for inflammation and immune function.

How to use this book: A guide to meal planning and recipes.

Welcome to "Lupus Diet Solutions: Proven Strategies to Heal Your Body with Anti-Inflammatory Recipes for Symptom Relief." This book is intended to serve as a comprehensive reference to learning how diet can affect your health and effectively manage lupus symptoms.

Navigating the Chapters: Each chapter of this book is designed to provide you with valuable information and practical tools for incorporating an anti-inflammatory diet into your daily life. You'll find detailed explanations of what foods to eat, what to avoid, and how to prepare balanced meals that nourish your body.

In the meal planning section, you'll find templates and strategies to make it easier to plan and prepare meals, which is one of the most difficult aspects of starting a new diet. We'll also go over the importance of grocery shopping with intention, stocking your pantry with anti-inflammatory staples, and batch cooking to save time during busy weeks.

In this book, you'll learn how to prepare meals that not only taste great but also provide your body with the nutrients it requires to thrive. The recipes in this book are designed to be both tasty and nutritious, and they range from vibrant breakfast options to hearty dinners and satisfying snacks.

Inspiration and Support: Living with lupus can feel isolating, but you are not alone. Throughout the book, you will find testimonials and stories from others who have gone through similar experiences, which can provide encouragement and a sense of community as you embark on your healing journey.

While diet is an important part of managing lupus, this book also emphasizes the importance of a holistic approach to health. You'll find sections dedicated to stress management techniques, the significance of hydration, and the necessity of quality sleep, all of which play a vital role in overall wellness and symptom management. Keep in mind that the journey toward managing lupus through diet is a personal one.

Let's investigate the transforming power of food together, and see how choosing informed dietary choices may lead to a brighter, healthier tomorrow.

Chapter 1: The Lupus Diet Essentials

An Overview of Anti-Inflammatory Foods

Understanding the impact of diet on inflammation is crucial in managing lupus. An anti-inflammatory diet can be a lifestyle change that improves overall well-being, reduces symptoms, and helps prevent flare-ups. This chapter will delve into the essence of anti-inflammatory foods, detailing what to eat and why they are important in your daily life.

Inflammation is a natural immune system response, but in autoimmune conditions like lupus, it can become overactive, causing tissue damage and increased symptoms. An anti-inflammatory diet focuses on minimizing foods that promote inflammation and maximizing those that combat it. By selecting the right foods, you can help regulate inflammation and support your body's healing processes.

Healing Foods: What to Eat

When it comes to food, variety and quality are important. The following categories of healing foods are essential for developing a well-rounded anti-inflammatory diet that can make a real impact in your health.

Organic, unprocessed foods

One of the most effective ways to begin an anti-inflammatory diet is to choose organic, unprocessed foods. Because organic foods are grown without the use of synthetic pesticides and fertilizers, they are free of potentially harmful chemicals that can cause inflammation.

Additionally, unprocessed foods retain their natural nutrients, making them more beneficial to your health.

Why Choose Organic?

Reduced Chemical Exposure: Because conventional farming frequently uses toxic pesticides that might linger on fruits and vegetables, going organic lowers your exposure to these chemicals.

Nutrient Density: Studies show that organic produce may include more antioxidants, vitamins, and minerals than conventionally farmed foods, all of which are important for your immune system and overall health.

Sustainability: Organic farming practices are frequently more sustainable, fostering a healthier ecosystem that improves your health in the long term.

Incorporate a variety of organic foods into your diet, focusing on whole grains, legumes, nuts, seeds, and a rainbow of fruits and vegetables. This strategy will ensure that you obtain a wide range of nutrients that contribute to inflammation reduction and immune response enhancement.

Raw and cooked vegetables

Vegetables are the foundation of any anti-inflammatory diet, and both raw and cooked types provide distinct health advantages. Fresh vegetables are high in vitamins, minerals, and antioxidants, all of which play an important role in reducing inflammation.

Raw vegetables:

Raw veggies, such as bell peppers, carrots, and cucumbers, are wonderful raw snacks that provide fiber and hydration while also preserving enzymes and minerals that can be lost during cooking.

Detoxification: Many raw vegetables, such as cruciferous vegetables like kale, broccoli, and Brussels sprouts, include substances that help the liver's detoxification activities, which are essential for treating autoimmune disorders like lupus.

Cooked vegetables:

Cooking certain vegetables, such as tomatoes, carrots, and spinach, might improve nutritional availability. Cooking tomatoes, for example, enhances the bioavailability of lycopene, an antioxidant that can help reduce inflammation.

Cooking can also make veggies easier to digest, allowing your body to absorb their nutrients more effectively. Steaming or roasting vegetables preserves their nutritional content while improving their flavor.

Incorporate a variety of raw and cooked veggies into your meals; try making colorful salads or roasted vegetable medleys that not only taste good but also provide a variety of nutrients that are beneficial to your health.

Fresh Fruits and their Benefits

Fruits are nature's sweet, and they play an important part in an anti-inflammatory diet. Fruits are high in vitamins, minerals, and antioxidants, which can help counteract oxidative stress and reduce inflammation in the body.

Best fruits for lupus:

Berries: Blueberries, strawberries, and raspberries are particularly strong in antioxidants known as flavonoids, which have been shown to lower inflammation and boost immunological function. They make fantastic snacks, oatmeal toppings, or smoothie additions.

Citrus fruits, such as oranges, lemons, and grapefruits, are strong in vitamin C, which is vital for immune health. Citrus also contains antioxidants, which can help reduce inflammation and strengthen your body's defenses.

Apples and pears are abundant in fiber and polyphenols, which have anti-inflammatory effects; eating the skin adds nutrients and benefits.

Aim to include a variety of fruits in your diet, experimenting with seasonal options to keep your meals new and exciting. Smoothies, fruit salads, and snacks are all terrific ways to incorporate these nutritious foods into your daily routine.

Wild-caught Fish and Omega-3 Fatty Acids

When it comes to protein sources, wild-caught fish stands out as a superfood for individuals managing lupus. Fish, particularly fatty fish like salmon, mackerel, sardines, and trout, are rich in omega-3 fatty acids, which are known to have potent anti-inflammatory qualities.

Advantages of Omega-3 Fatty Acids:

Reduced Inflammation: Omega-3 fatty acids have been found to lessen the synthesis of inflammatory chemicals in the body, which can lead to fewer symptoms and a higher quality of life for lupus patients.

People with lupus are more likely to develop cardiovascular disease, thus heart-healthy meals such as omega-3-rich fish are essential for general health.

Omega-3s also help with cognitive function, which is useful considering the cognitive issues that some lupus patients suffer.

Incorporate wild-caught fish into your diet at least two to three times each week. Grilling, baking, or sautéing fish with healthy fats like olive oil may produce a delicious and nutritious meal that promotes your health.

Probiotic-rich foods help maintain a healthy gut flora, which is critical for strengthening the immune system and lowering inflammation. Gut health is important for overall health, especially for people suffering from autoimmune diseases.

Top probiotic foods:

Fermented Dairy: Yogurt and kefir are excellent sources of probiotics; look for kinds with live active cultures and no added sugars for best benefits.

Fermented Vegetables: Sauerkraut, kimchi, and pickles created from natural fermentation include beneficial bacteria that promote intestinal health.

Tempeh and Miso: These soy-based meals are high in probiotics and also include protein and other necessary elements.

Incorporating probiotic-rich foods into your diet helps improve digestion, increase nutrient absorption, and promote immune function. Aim to include these items on a regular basis, whether in smoothies, salads, or side dishes.

Bone Broth's Advantages

Bone broth is a traditional dish that has witnessed a resurgence in popularity due to its multiple health advantages. Made by simmering animal bones, this nutrient-rich broth is full with minerals, amino acids, and collagen.

Benefits of Bone Broth:

Supports Joint Health: The collagen in bone broth can help strengthen joints and reduce pain and inflammation, making it especially beneficial for lupus patients who frequently encounter joint problems.

Bone broth has been shown to improve gut health by increasing gut lining integrity, which is necessary for controlling inflammation and immunological responses.

Nutrient-dense: It contains vitamins and minerals that can nourish your body and promote overall wellness.

Incorporate bone broth into your meals by sipping it warm or using it as a base for soups and stews. This nutritious liquid can become a soothing staple in your anti-inflammatory diet.

Herbs, spices, and tea

Herbs and spices are not only tasty, but they also have anti-inflammatory properties. Many herbs and spices include bioactive components that can reduce inflammation and improve general health.

Strong Anti-Inflammatory Herbs & Spices:

Turmeric, a vivid yellow spice that contains curcumin, a potent anti-inflammatory component, can be added to soups, smoothies, or golden milk to provide an extra health boost.

Ginger, known for its anti-nausea characteristics, also has anti-inflammatory effects; use it in teas, smoothies, or stir-fries to add flavor and health benefits.

Garlic is a natural immune booster that contains sulfur compounds that help reduce inflammation. Fresh garlic can be used in cooking to enhance flavor and health benefits.

Cinnamon: This sweet spice can help decrease blood sugar levels and has anti-inflammatory qualities; sprinkle it on oatmeal, yogurt, or baked goods for a tasty health boost.

In addition to herbs and spices, consider drinking herbal teas such as chamomile, peppermint, or green tea, which contain antioxidants that can help reduce inflammation while also providing hydration.

Incorporating anti-inflammatory foods into your diet is a powerful way to take control of your health and manage lupus symptoms. Focusing on organic, unprocessed foods, fresh fruits and vegetables, omega-3 fatty acids from fish, probiotic-rich foods, bone broth, and beneficial herbs and spices, you can create a nutritious diet that supports your body's healing processes.

As you continue on your path, let this chapter serve as your guide to selecting and preparing the meals that will help you thrive in the face of lupus. Keep in mind that even minor changes in your diet can result in huge improvements in your general well-being.

Chapter 2: Foods To Avoid

In this chapter, we'll look at the various inflammatory foods that can aggravate symptoms and disrupt your healing journey. Eliminating or significantly reducing these foods from your diet can help you improve your overall well-being and reduce the frequency and intensity of lupus symptoms.

Understanding Inflammatory Foods

The term "inflammatory foods" refers to those items that can trigger or exacerbate inflammation in the body. Consuming these foods can lead to a cascade of reactions that may worsen lupus symptoms, causing fatigue, joint pain, and digestive issues, among other things. Knowing the key offenders is essential for anyone committed to improving their health and managing their condition effectively.

Transfats and hydrogenated oils

Trans fats are one of the most dangerous ingredients found in many processed foods. These fats, which are often listed on labels as partially hydrogenated oils, are created by adding hydrogen to liquid vegetable oils, turning them into a solid form. This process makes trans fats particularly stable for frying and gives processed foods a longer shelf life, but it comes at a high cost to your health.

Why Should I Avoid Trans Fats?

Trans fats have been found in studies to increase inflammation in the body, which is especially worrying for lupus patients because chronic inflammation can worsen symptoms and contribute to long-term health concerns.

Heart Health Risks: Trans fats have been associated to an increased risk of heart disease, which is especially problematic for lupus patients, who are already predisposed to cardiovascular problems.

Trans fat consumption has a negative impact on lipid profiles, increasing LDL (bad) cholesterol levels while decreasing HDL (good) cholesterol levels, contributing to inflammation and heart disease.

To avoid trans fats, stay away from processed snacks, baked products, fried foods, and anything with partially hydrogenated oils. Always check the nutrition label for trans fat content, and choose healthy fats like olive oil, avocado oil, or coconut oil, which have anti-inflammatory properties.

Refined carbs and gluten

Refined carbs, such as white bread, pastries, and sugary cereals, are depleted of important nutrients and fiber during processing. This lack of nutritional value might cause blood sugar increases and inflammation.

The Problem With Refined Carbs:

Insulin Resistance: Excessive consumption of refined carbohydrates can cause insulin resistance, a condition in which the body's cells no longer respond to insulin properly. This resistance can worsen inflammation and is frequently associated to autoimmune illnesses like lupus.

Weight Gain: Refined carbohydrates are frequently calorie-dense but nutrient-deficient, resulting in weight gain and obesity, which are extra pressures on the body and can exacerbate lupus symptoms.

Gluten Sensitivity: For some people with lupus, gluten—a protein found in wheat, barley, and rye—can be an issue in their diet. While not everyone with lupus is gluten-sensitive, those who are may have increased inflammation and intestinal pain after consuming it.

Why Go Gluten-Free?

Reduced Inflammation: For gluten-sensitive people, eliminating it can result in considerable reductions in inflammation, fewer flare-ups, and an overall improvement in well-being.

Better Digestive Health: A gluten-free diet can boost gut health by removing possible irritants and encouraging a healthy microbiota.

To limit your intake of processed carbohydrates and gluten, go for whole grains such as quinoa, brown rice, and oats. These options give fiber and nutrition while avoiding the inflammatory consequences of processed grains.

Conventional Dairy Products

Dairy products might be a mixed bag for people with lupus. While some people can tolerate dairy without problems, others may find that typical dairy worsens their symptoms.

The Issue with Conventional Dairy:

Hormonal Influences: Many dairy products are derived from cows that have been treated with hormones and antibiotics, which can disturb your body's hormonal balance and increase inflammation.

Lactose Intolerance: Lactose intolerance is widespread, and eating dairy products can cause bloating, gas, and digestive discomfort in lupus patients, increasing fatigue and malaise.

What about alternatives? If you dislike conventional dairy, try almond milk, coconut yogurt, or lactose-free dairy products. These alternatives can deliver comparable textures and flavors without the inflammatory consequences associated with traditional dairy.

Processed and Fast Food

The ease of processed and fast foods frequently comes at a cost. While they may save time and effort in meal preparation, they are frequently filled with toxic components that can worsen inflammation.

Why are processed foods problematic?

Sugars and salts: Many processed foods have added sugars, preservatives, and trans fats, all of which can cause inflammation and contribute to chronic diseases.

Low nutritional value: Fast foods are often deficient in critical nutrients and antioxidants required to battle inflammation and boost the immune system.

Healthier Alternatives: Instead of eating fast food, try meal preparing or using whole, fresh products to make meals at home. Focus on nutrient-dense foods that provide energy and nutrients without causing inflammation.

Nightshade Vegetables: Myths and Reality

Nightshade foods, such as tomatoes, potatoes, eggplants, and peppers, have earned a mixed reputation in the health world. Some feel certain meals can worsen inflammation, while others believe they are healthy.

The Myth: Some people believe that nightshades contain substances like solanine, which can cause inflammation. However, scientific evidence on this is conflicting.

The Reality:

Nutrient-dense: Nightshade vegetables are typically high in vitamins, minerals, and antioxidants. For many people, they might be a beneficial complement to an anti-inflammatory diet.

Individual Responses: The key is individual tolerance. While some people experience symptoms after eating nightshades, others do not. Listen to your body and find out what works best for you.

If you believe that nightshades are contributing to your symptoms, try avoiding them for a few weeks before gradually returning them to see how your body reacts.

Alcohol and the Effects on Lupus

For people with lupus, drinking alcohol can be a steep slope. While moderate alcohol use may not be harmful to everyone, it can have negative consequences for some lupus sufferers.

Potential Risks:

Inflammation: Alcohol can cause inflammation in the body, which is particularly dangerous for people who already have an autoimmune disorder.

Medication Interactions: Many lupus patients use medications that interact poorly with alcohol, potentially leading to increased side effects or decreased efficacy.

Dehydration: Alcohol can cause dehydration, and staying hydrated is essential for controlling lupus symptoms.

Making Informed Decisions: If you decide to drink alcohol, do so in moderation and check with your doctor to learn how it may affect your health and prescription regimen. Consider alternatives, such as herbal teas or non-alcoholic beverages, which can provide a pleasurable experience without causing inflammation.

Chapter 3: Menu Planning for Lupus

Living with lupus needs a conscientious attitude to eating, and meal planning is a valuable tool for properly managing your symptoms. By planning your meals ahead of time, you can ensure that you are constantly feeding your body anti-inflammatory nutrients while avoiding potential triggers. This chapter will walk you through the steps of establishing a personalized meal plan, including sample templates, grocery shopping advice, and techniques for batch cooking and meal preparing. With proper planning, you may make your eating habits a source of power and vigor.

Building Your Weekly Meal Plan

A well-structured meal plan promotes health while also saving you time and stress in the kitchen. Here's how to construct a food plan that is specific to your needs.

1. Assess your nutritional needs.

Before you start meal planning, you need first examine your nutritional needs. Consider the following.

Caloric intake varies depending on your exercise level and overall health. Consult a healthcare physician or a qualified dietician to establish your unique needs.

Macro and micronutrients: Achieve a balance of proteins, healthy fats, and carbohydrates. Aim to receive a range of vitamins and minerals from colorful fruits and vegetables.

2. Create a template.

A meal planning template might help to simplify the process. Here's a simple format to get you started:

Day's meals: breakfast, lunch, dinner, and snacks.

Monday: avocado toast with eggs, Quinoa salad with vegetables, grilled salmon with broccoli, almonds, and berries.

Tuesday meal options include a spinach smoothie, lentil soup with whole grain bread, chicken stir-fry with brown rice, carrot sticks, and hummus.

Wednesday's meals include oatmeal with chia seeds, Greek yogurt with nuts, zucchini noodles with marinara, and celery with almond butter.

Thursday meal options include scrambled eggs and spinach, tuna salad with mixed greens, stuffed bell peppers, and sliced apple with cheese.

Friday meal options include chia pudding with fruit, black bean tacos, baked sweet potato with quinoa, and air-popped popcorn.

Saturday's meal included almond flour pancakes, chicken Caesar salad, veggie curry with brown rice, and dark chocolate squares

Sunday meal options include smoothie bowl, grilled vegetable wrap, roasted chicken with vegetables, and mixed nuts.

3. Variety is key.

To avoid meal fatigue, include a variety of foods and recipes. Throughout the week, try to vary your protein sources (fish, poultry, legumes) and grains (quinoa, brown rice, farro). This not only makes your meals more fascinating, but it also assures you obtain a variety of nutrients.

4. Prepare for flexibility.

Life can be unpredictable, so incorporate some flexibility into your meal plan. Plan one or two "flex meals" per week in which you can use leftovers or eat out. Having a few quick, healthful dishes on hand for those hectic days might also help.

Sample Meal Planning Templates:

In addition to the weekly template supplied above, here are a few more alternatives to fit different interests or lifestyles:

Monthly Meal Planning Template

A monthly template might be a more comprehensive tool for those who wish to prepare ahead. Include seasonal ingredients and dishes that can be rotated throughout the month.

Grocery List Integration

Creating a grocery list based on your meal plan can help to streamline your shopping visits. To make your shopping experience more effective, organize the list by food groups (fruits, vegetables, proteins, grains, etc.).

Meal Preparation Specific Template

Consider including meal prep sections in your menu, indicating which dishes can be batch-cooked and stored for later. For example:

Day's Meal Preparation Notes

Monday: cook quinoa for the week.

Tuesday: Roast vegetables for salad.

Wednesday: Make a double batch of lentil soup.

Thursday: Prepare smoothie packs for breakfast.

Friday: Grill additional chicken for wraps.

By combining several templates and ideas, you can develop a meal planning system that works for you and keeps you on track with your nutritional objectives.

Tips For Grocery Shopping and Pantry Stocking

A grocery shopping approach might help you avoid impulsive purchases and stay on track with your meal plan. Here are some suggestions to make your buying experience smoother:

1. Shop the perimeter.

Grocery shops frequently display fresh vegetables, dairy, and meats around the perimeter, whereas processed commodities are typically located in the aisles. Begin your shopping in these exterior sections to load your cart with entire, nutritious foods before moving into the aisles.

2. Create a detailed list.

Before going to the supermarket, make a complete shopping list based on your food plan. Group things by category to save time while shopping and reduce the likelihood of forgetting important elements.

3. Choose seasonal and local foods.

Purchasing seasonal produce not only benefits local farmers, but it also assures that you are receiving the freshest products. Seasonal fruits and vegetables are more cheap and tasty.

4. Stock up on staples.

Maintain a well-stocked pantry with vital staples, such as:

Whole grains (quinoa, brown rice, and oatmeal)

Canned beans and legumes

Healthy oils (olive and avocado oil)

Spices & herbs

Frozen fruits and vegetables for fast dinners.

5. Read Labels Carefully.

When purchasing packaged foods, be sure to read the nutrition labels. Look for items with few ingredients and avoid those that contain extra sweets, trans fats, or preservatives. To avoid pesticides and additives, opt for organic products wherever feasible.

Batch Cooking and Meal Preparation Strategies

Batch cooking and meal preparing can help you save time during hectic weeks while also ensuring that you have healthful meals on hand. Here are some ways to make the procedure more efficient:

1. Choose a Cooking Day.

Set aside a specific day each week (such as Sunday) for batch cooking. Use this time to make several meals or components, such as cereals, proteins, and vegetables.

2. Prepare versatile ingredients.

Cook huge quantities of flexible ingredients that may be used in several meals. For example, roast a large tray of mixed vegetables that may be used in salads, wraps, or as a side dish all week.

3. Invest in quality containers.

Using high-quality airtight containers is essential for keeping your meals fresh. Choose glass or BPA-free plastic containers that may be easily stacked in the refrigerator or freezer.

4. Label everything.

Label your containers with the meal's name and date of preparation. This allows you to keep track of freshness and eat meals before they deteriorate.

5. Create a freezer inventory.

If you batch prepare and store meals, maintain a running list of what you have in the freezer. This can help you reduce waste and make meal planning easier.

Chapter 4: Recipes for Relief.

Eating to relieve lupus symptoms entails consuming a wide range of delectable, anti-inflammatory foods that nourish both the body and the soul. This chapter is dedicated to providing you with a variety of appealing dishes, ranging from energizing breakfasts to filling dinners and delicious snacks. Each dish is intended to not only satisfy your taste buds but also provide the restorative benefits your body need. Let's look at some delectable foods that can help you manage lupus.

Breakfast Ideas:

A nutritious meal sets the tone for the rest of the day, giving you the energy and nutrients you need to face the demands of daily life. Here are some excellent breakfast ideas high in anti-inflammatory components.

Anti-inflammatory Smoothies

Smoothies are a quick and adaptable way to start your morning. They allow you to combine a variety of anti-inflammatory components into a single, tasty beverage. Here's a powerful recipe.

Berry Spinach Smoothie

Ingredients:

1 cup of fresh spinach.

1/2 cup mixed berries, such as blueberries, strawberries, or raspberries

1/2 banana.

1 tablespoon flaxseeds.

1 cup of unsweetened almond milk.

One teaspoon honey (optional)

Instructions:

Combine all items in a blender.

Blend until smooth, adjusting the thickness with extra almond milk as needed.

Pour in a glass and enjoy!

Benefits: This smoothie contains antioxidants from the berries, omega-3 fatty acids from flaxseeds, and a variety of vitamins from spinach, all of which can help to reduce inflammation.

Overnight Oats With Superfoods

Overnight oats are ideal for hectic mornings. They're simple to make, versatile with a variety of toppings, and high in fiber.

Chia Seeds Overnight Oats

Ingredients:

1/2 cup rolled oats.

1 tablespoon of chia seeds.

1 cup of unsweetened almond milk.

1/2 teaspoon of cinnamon.

One tablespoon maple syrup.

Fresh fruits and nuts for topping.

Instructions:

In a jar or bowl, combine the rolled oats, chia seeds, almond milk, cinnamon, and maple syrup.

Stir thoroughly, cover, and refrigerate overnight.

In the morning, top with your favorite toppings, such as sliced bananas, walnuts, or berries.

Benefits: The combination of oats and chia seeds provides a significant amount of fiber and protein, boosting digestive health and balancing blood sugar levels.

Lunch Options:

To maintain your energy levels, midday meals should be both nourishing and satisfying. Here are two healthy lunch options that are high in taste and nutrients.

Nourishing Salads with Grain Bowls

Salads and grain bowls are quite versatile, allowing you to combine ingredients based on what you have on hand.

Quinoa & Kale Salad

Ingredients:

1 cup cooked quinoa.

2 cups chopped kale.

1/2 cup cherry tomatoes (halved)

1/4 cup diced cucumber.

1/4 cup feta cheese (optional).

2 tablespoons olive oil.

Juice from 1 lemon

Add salt and pepper to taste.

Instructions:

In a large bowl, combine the cooked quinoa, kale, cherry tomatoes, cucumber, and feta cheese.

In a small bowl, combine olive oil, lemon juice, salt, and pepper.

Drizzle the dressing over the salad and mix well.

Benefits: This salad is high in antioxidants, fiber, and healthy fats, making it an excellent choice for lowering inflammation.

Soups and Stews Full of Nutrients

A substantial soup or stew may be both warming and healthful, particularly during the colder months.

Turmeric Lentil Soup

Ingredients:

Angela. O.

1 cup, washed lentils

1 onion, chopped

Two carrots, chopped

Two celery stalks, chopped

4 garlic cloves, minced

1 tablespoon of turmeric powder.

6 cups veggie broth.

Add salt and pepper to taste.

Fresh cilantro for garnish.

Instructions:

In a large pot, cook the onion, carrots, and celery until tender.

Cook for another minute until the garlic and turmeric are aromatic.

Stir in the lentils and vegetable broth. Bring to a boil, then reduce the heat and simmer for 30 minutes.

Season with salt and pepper, then garnish with cilantro before serving.

Benefits: Turmeric is known for its anti-inflammatory effects, making this soup ideal for lupus patients.

Dinner Favorites

Dinner is an opportunity to provide your body with nutritious ingredients. Here are some ideas for tasty and nutritious dinners.

Healthy Protein Sources and Sides

Consuming lean proteins is vital for muscle regeneration and overall health.

Baked Salmon and Asparagus

Ingredients:

Two salmon fillets.

One bunch of asparagus, trimmed

2 tablespoons olive oil.

One lemon, sliced

Add salt and pepper to taste.

Instructions:

Preheat the oven to 400 °F (200 °C).

On a baking sheet, arrange the salmon fillets and asparagus.

Drizzle with olive oil, then season with salt and pepper. Top the salmon with lemon wedges.

Bake for 15-20 minutes, or until the salmon is thoroughly cooked and easily flaked.

Benefits: Salmon is high in omega-3 fatty acids, which might help reduce inflammation. Asparagus offers additional vitamins and antioxidants.

Creative Vegetable Dishes

Vegetables are essential components of any anti-inflammatory diet. Be inventive with your preparations to make them more enticing.

Roasted Vegetable Medley.

Ingredients:

1 zucchini, sliced

<u>**Angela. O.**</u>

1 bell pepper, diced

1 cup of broccoli florets.

1 cup of cauliflower florets.

2 tablespoons olive oil.

1 teaspoon of garlic powder.

Add salt and pepper to taste.

Instructions:

Preheat the oven to 425° Fahrenheit (220° Celsius).

Mix all vegetables in a bowl with olive oil, garlic powder, salt, and pepper.

Spread out on a baking sheet and roast for 20-25 minutes, until soft and slightly browned.

Benefits: This bright combination is high in vitamins and minerals that promote immune function and general health.

Snack and Dessert

Healthy snacks and desserts can fulfill your appetites while meeting your nutritional needs.

Healthy Snack Ideas

Snacking can be beneficial to your anti-inflammatory journey if you choose the correct foods.

Spicy Roasted Chickpeas

Ingredients:

1 can of chickpeas, drained and rinsed

1 tablespoon of olive oil.

1 teaspoon of paprika.

1/2 teaspoon of cayenne pepper.

Salt to taste.

Instructions:

Preheat the oven to 400 °F (200 °C).

Pat chickpeas dry before tossing with olive oil, paprika, cayenne, and salt.

Spread on a baking sheet and roast for 20-30 minutes, until crispy.

Chickpeas are high in protein and fiber, which helps you stay full and energized.

Delicious Dessert Recipes Without Refined Sugar

You do not have to give up dessert to keep a healthy diet. Here's a delicious recipe that is organically sweetened.

Coconut Chia Pudding

Ingredients:

1/2 cup chia seeds.

2 cups coconut milk, unsweetened

1 tablespoon honey or maple syrup.

Fresh fruits for topping (e.g., mango and berries)

Instructions:

In a mixing bowl, add chia seeds, coconut milk, and maple syrup. Stir thoroughly.

Cover and refrigerate for at least 4 hours or overnight to thicken.

Serve topped with fresh fruit.

Benefits: This pudding contains omega-3 fatty acids and fiber, making it a healthy way to satisfy your sweet taste.

Chapter 5: Lifestyle Changes to Support Healing.

Living with Lupus brings distinct problems that go beyond the clinical signs of the disease. While a nutritious diet is essential for managing inflammation and maintaining overall health, making lifestyle changes can dramatically improve your healing process. In this chapter, we will look at key lifestyle adjustments that can help you manage lupus more effectively. We'll talk about stress management tactics, the significance of staying hydrated, and sleep hygiene practices that can help your body and mind rest and recover.

Stress Management Techniques

Stress can increase lupus symptoms and cause flares, therefore good stress management is critical. By combining mindfulness techniques and physical activity into your daily routine, you can create a sense of calm and resilience.

Mindfulness and Relaxation Practices

Mindfulness is the practice of remaining in the present moment and monitoring your thoughts without judgment. It has been demonstrated to relieve stress, boost mood, and promote general well-being. Here are some mindfulness methods to include in your daily routine:

Set aside time each day for meditation. Find a quiet place, close your eyes, and concentrate on your breathing. To get started, use guided meditation applications or watch videos. Aim for 10-20 minutes per day to receive the benefits.

Deep breathing exercises help to relax the nervous system and relieve tension. Use this technique:

Sit or lie comfortably.

Inhale deeply through your nose for a count of four to fill your lungs.

Hold your breath for a count of four.

Exhale slowly through your mouth for a count of four.

Repeat for five cycles.

Progressive Muscle Relaxation: This technique consists of tensing and relaxing various muscle groups in your body. It can help you become more conscious of physical stress and promote relaxation:

Begin with your toes, strain for five seconds, then relax.

Work your way up to your head by starting with your calves, then your thighs, and so on.

Yoga: Adding mild yoga to your program can help reduce stress and improve flexibility. Many online platforms provide classes designed specifically for those with chronic diseases, focusing on gentle movements and breathwork.

The Role of Physical Activity

Regular physical activity benefits both physical and mental health. Endorphins are natural mood boosters that are released after exercise. Here are some methods to incorporate physical activity into your lifestyle:

Low-Impact Exercises: Activities such as walking, swimming, and cycling can provide cardiovascular benefits without putting undue effort on the body. Aim to complete at least 150 minutes of moderate-intensity aerobic activity every week.

Strength Training: Incorporating strength training activities can help to enhance muscle strength and overall health. Concentrate on low-resistance workouts with body weight or resistance bands, aiming for two sessions each week.

Listen to Your Body: It's critical to monitor how your body reacts to exercise. If you feel exhausted or in pain, change your routine or take a day off. The idea is to strike a balance that suits you.

Hydration: Importance and Best Practices.

Staying hydrated is essential for everyone, but it is especially important for those with lupus. Proper hydration promotes biological functioning, aids in detoxification, and can alleviate symptoms such as weariness and joint pain.

Importance of Hydration

Maintaining bodily functions: Water is required for digestion, circulation, and temperature regulation. It helps to provide nutrients to cells and eliminate waste from the body.

Managing Symptoms: Dehydration can worsen fatigue and joint discomfort. Staying hydrated can help to ease these sensations, leaving you feeling more energized and comfortable.

Preventing Flare-Ups: Proper hydration may also help lessen the likelihood of flare-ups, as dehydration can increase the stress on your body.

Best Practices for Hydration

Aim for Adequate Water Intake: While individual hydration requirements differ, a basic rule is to consume at least eight 8-ounce glasses of water per day. Adjust the amount based on your exercise level, climate, and overall health.

Incorporate Hydrating Foods: Many fruits and vegetables are high in water and can help you stay hydrated. Include cucumbers, watermelon, oranges, and leafy greens in your diet.

Limit Dehydrating Beverages: Caffeine and alcohol can cause dehydration. If you consume these beverages, make sure to drink plenty of water. Herbal teas are an excellent option, delivering hydration without the dehydrating effects of caffeine.

Listen to Your Body: Pay close attention to your thirst signals and the color of your urine. A pale yellow pee often indicates appropriate hydration, however darker urine may indicate a need for extra fluids.

Sleep Hygiene: Creating a Restful Environment

Quality sleep is essential for recovery and general health. People with lupus frequently have sleep difficulties, which can lead to exhaustion and aggravate symptoms. Practicing proper sleep hygiene can dramatically enhance your sleep quality.

Creating Restful Environments

Create a Sleep Schedule: Aim to go to bed and wake up at the same time every day, including weekends. This constancy can help regulate your body's internal clock, allowing you to go asleep more easily and wake up feeling refreshed.

Design a Sleep-Inducing setting: Create a relaxing bedroom setting. Keep the room dark, chilly, and silent. Consider utilizing blackout curtains, white noise machines, or earplugs as needed.

Limit Screen Time Before Bed: Blue light from screens might interfere with melatonin production, making it difficult to fall asleep. Aim to switch off electronic gadgets at least an hour before bed. Instead, consider reading a book, keeping a notebook, or doing relaxation exercises.

Establish a Relaxing Bedtime ritual: A peaceful pre-sleep ritual helps alert your body that it is time to unwind. Gentle stretching, meditation, and taking a warm bath can all help you relax.

Evaluate Your Mattress and Pillows: Investing in a comfortable mattress and supportive pillows can significantly improve your sleep quality. When selecting the appropriate pillows, keep your favorite sleeping position in mind.

Limit Naps During the Day: While short naps might help with exhaustion, extended or inconsistent naps can disrupt nocturnal sleep. If you need to nap, schedule 20-30 minutes earlier in the day.

Integrating these lifestyle modifications can have a significant impact on your lupus treatment. You may improve your general well-being and help your body repair by controlling stress with mindfulness and physical activity, prioritizing hydration, and creating restful sleep settings. Remember, the route to wellness is a marathon, not a sprint. Take it one step at a time, be gentle to yourself, and enjoy your minor triumphs along the road.

Chapter 6: Working With Healthcare Professionals

Navigating life with Lupus is a difficult process that necessitates a comprehensive approach to healthcare. While food and lifestyle modifications are important in controlling an autoimmune disorder, working closely with healthcare specialists can help you better understand lupus and make more informed decisions. In this chapter, we'll go over the importance of working with dietitians and nutritionists, monitoring symptoms and dietary effects, and getting frequent medical check-ups.

Working with dietitians and nutritionists

Dietitians and nutritionists are invaluable resources in your lupus management journey. They have specialist knowledge of how food affects the body, particularly inflammatory diseases. Working with these professionals can help you create a nutritional plan that is tailored to your specific needs.

Understanding Their Roles

Registered dietitians (RDs) are nutrition specialists who have met certain educational criteria and passed a national exam. They can create nutritional recommendations according to your health goals, medical history, and preferences.

Nutritionists: Although the term "nutritionist" is less regulated, many nutritionists have a thorough understanding of dietary patterns. They can provide advice on making healthier food choices, meal planning, and lifestyle changes.

How to Work with Dietitians and Nutritionists?

Assess Your Needs: Before consulting with a dietitian or nutritionist, consider your individual dietary requirements, health problems, and lifestyle choices. Are there any specific symptoms you want to address? Have you have any food allergies or intolerances? Making a list of questions can help direct your talk.

Set Specific Goals: Discuss your health objectives during your initial visit. A dietitian or nutritionist can build a personalized plan to support your goals of reducing inflammation, managing fatigue, or improving your general well-being.

Regular Follow-ups: Schedule follow-up sessions to track your progress and change your diet as needed. These meetings allow you to share any issues you may be facing and receive additional support.

Keep an open mind: Be willing to test new foods and nutritional ideas. A dietician may expose you to anti-inflammatory foods or advise cooking methods you've never tried before.

Seek Evidence-Based Advice: Make sure your healthcare provider's suggestions are evidence-based. A well-informed dietitian or nutritionist will make recommendations based on current research.

Monitor Symptoms and Dietary Impact

Understanding how certain foods affect your symptoms is critical for successful lupus management. Keeping a careful record of your dietary consumption and symptoms might help you detect patterns and make informed nutritional decisions.

Keep a food journal.

A food journal is a useful tool for recording what you eat and how it impacts your health. Here is how to start:

Log Your Meals: Record everything you eat and drink, including portion sizes and preparation methods. Make sure you bring food and beverages.

Symptoms: Take note of any symptoms you have throughout the day, such as weariness, joint discomfort, skin rashes, or digestive problems. Include the timing of these symptoms to assist establish a link between food and reactions.

Identify trends: After a few weeks of keeping a food journal, go through your entries and look for trends. Are there certain foods that cause flare-ups or symptoms? Are there any goods that appear to ease discomfort? This information can help you make informed food choices and have talks with healthcare providers.

Bring your food journal to appointments with your dietician, nutritionist, or doctor. It can offer useful insights for developing a personalized management strategy.

Recognizing Dietary Triggers

Each person with lupus may react differently to specific meals. Processed sweets, trans fats, and gluten are common inflammatory foods, but you may also experience discomfort from other substances. Pay close attention to your body's signals and modify your diet accordingly.

The Importance of Regular Medical Checkups

Regular medical checkups are essential for good lupus care. These appointments allow your healthcare team to monitor your condition, assess therapy efficacy, and make any required changes to your management plan.

Establishing a Healthcare Team

Lupus is often managed using a multidisciplinary approach. Your healthcare team may include the following:

A rheumatologist is an autoimmune disease expert who plays an important role in detecting and treating lupus. They can prescribe drugs, track disease progression, and offer advice on how to manage symptoms.

Primary Care Physician: Your primary care physician may oversee your overall health, conduct routine screenings, and address any non-lupus health concerns.

Dietitian/Nutritionist: As previously stated, these specialists can assist you in developing a diet that promotes good health and addresses lupus-related difficulties.

Mental Health Professional: Living with a chronic condition can have a negative impact on mental health. Working with a therapist or counselor can help with emotional support and coping strategies.

Why Regular Check-Ups Matter

Monitoring Disease Progression: Lupus can impact numerous organ systems, and symptoms may alter over time. Regular check-ups help your healthcare team to monitor your condition, identify changes, and adapt treatment plans accordingly.

Evaluating Treatment Effectiveness: If you are taking medications to treat lupus symptoms, your doctor will need to keep track of how you respond to them. Regular check-ups can assist determine whether your drugs are working or if changes are needed.

Preventing problems: Lupus can cause a variety of problems, including cardiovascular disease, kidney damage, and infection. Routine tests and evaluations can help detect any problems early on, allowing for prompt solutions.

Updating Health Information: Your healthcare practitioner may need to review your medical history, prescriptions, and allergies at each appointment. Keeping your records up to date ensures you receive the best possible treatment.

Developing a Supportive Relationship: Regular check-ups help you establish a rapport with your healthcare team. Feeling at ease addressing your issues can lead to more effective treatment and improved health outcomes.

Collaboration with healthcare experts is critical for effectively controlling lupus. You may take control of your health by working closely with dietitians and nutritionists, evaluating the effects of your food on your symptoms, and scheduling frequent medical check-ups. Remember that you are not alone in this journey; a supportive healthcare team can assist you negotiate the difficulties of lupus.

Chapter Seven: Personal Stories and Testimonials

One of the most significant resources available for managing lupus is other people's lived experiences. Personal stories and testimonies not only inspire and bring hope, but they also demonstrate the practical advantages of dietary adjustments. In this chapter, we will look at real-life experiences of lupus patients, how dietary changes have made a huge difference in their lives, and recommendations from individuals who have successfully navigated this difficult condition.

Real-Life Experiences of Lupus Patients

Samantha's journey: from struggle to strength.

<u>Angela. O.</u>

Samantha was diagnosed with lupus at the age of 27, when she thought her life had just begun. As a runner and outdoor enthusiast, the diagnosis hit her hard. Samantha initially experienced terrible weariness, joint discomfort, and skin rashes, forcing her to cut back on things she enjoyed. She frequently felt dissatisfied and overwhelmed, unable to keep up with the demands of daily living.

During her darkest times, a friend connected her to a lupus support group, where she heard stories about how others had found relief through dietary adjustments. Samantha was inspired and resolved to take action. She started her journey by cutting out processed foods, sugar, and gluten from her diet and replacing them with whole, organic foods.

Samantha observed a significant transformation after several months of following her new eating habits. Her energy levels improved, her joint pain subsided, and she began running again. What seemed like a distant goal became a reality when she finished her first 5K since being diagnosed.

Samantha's experience reminds us that with determination and the correct tools, we can recover control of our health.

Mark's Transformation: The Power Of Nutrition

Mark, a 40-year-old father of two, had lupus for more than a decade before finding the link between nutrition and symptom control. He initially relied extensively on medication to treat his difficulties, but he frequently suffered side effects that made him feel worse than before. After after thorough study, Mark discovered the value of an anti-inflammatory diet and decided to experiment with his nutrition.

He began by including more fruits and vegetables in his diet, focusing on antioxidant-rich foods such as berries, leafy greens, and cruciferous vegetables. Mark also added wild-caught salmon to his diet, increasing his omega-3 consumption, and started drinking bone broth for its healing effects.

Within a few weeks, Mark observed substantial changes. His energy levels increased, and he felt more alert and concentrated all day. He shared his newfound knowledge with his family, inspiring them to make healthy food choices as well. They now enjoy making meals together and have made it a family ritual to prepare Sunday dinners using wholesome food.

Mark's story demonstrates how dietary changes may spread throughout a family, promoting a better lifestyle for all members.

How Dietary Changes Made A Difference

Samantha and Mark's tales highlight a frequent feature among lupus patients: dietary adjustments can lead to significant improvements in symptoms and overall well-being. But what does it look like in practice? Here are some important features of how dietary modifications have helped many people:

Reduced Inflammation: Many patients claim that eating anti-inflammatory foods like turmeric, ginger, and fatty fish has helped with joint pain and swelling. These foods include anti-inflammatory chemicals, which can provide relief that drugs alone cannot.

Increased Energy Levels: Switching to a nutrient-dense whole-foods diet can boost your energy levels. Patients frequently report that removing processed sugars and refined carbohydrates minimizes energy crashes and allows them to feel more balanced throughout the day.

Improved Digestive Health: Many lupus patients have found that eating probiotic-rich foods like yogurt and fermented vegetables is beneficial. Improved gut health can boost the immune system and help regulate systemic inflammation.

Mental Clarity and Mood Stability: A nutrient-dense diet benefits both brain health and emotional well-being. Many lupus patients report feeling less anxious and depressed after eating nutritious foods, suggesting the strong link between diet and mental health.

Empowerment and Control: Making informed dietary decisions empowers lupus sufferers. Understanding the effects of food on the body enables people to take an active role in controlling their health, resulting in enhanced confidence and resilience.

Tips from Those Who Have Been There.

The road of managing lupus through dietary adjustments is unique to each individual. However, individuals who have successfully traversed this path have given useful suggestions and observations. Here are some strategies to consider.

Start Slowly: Switching to a new diet might be stressful. Many lupus sufferers recommend starting with minor changes, such as introducing a new vegetable to meals or swapping a sugary snack for a piece of fruit. The gradual introduction of new meals provides for a more sustainable strategy.

Experiment and Listen to Your Body: Each person with lupus reacts differently to certain meals. Keep a food log to see how different foods affect your symptoms. This will aid in identifying triggers and developing a specific eating plan that is effective for you.

Find Support: Participating in support groups or online communities can help you feel encouraged and motivated. Sharing experiences with those who understand the complexities of lupus can be extremely empowering and educational.

Cooking may be a therapeutic release, and trying new recipes can make healthy eating more enjoyable. Experimenting with different spices, herbs, and cooking methods may turn basic foods into delectable dinners.

Prioritize Meal Planning: Making time to plan meals and snacks will help you avoid the temptation to grab for processed foods. Consider setting up one day every week to prepare meals ahead of time, which can help you stick to your nutritional goals.

Celebrate Progress: Recognize and celebrate your accomplishments, no matter how minor. Whether you've successfully removed a trigger food or discovered a new dish, acknowledging your accomplishments helps boost motivation and commitment.

Personal tales and testimonies from lupus patients demonstrate the dramatic influence that dietary modifications have on symptom management and overall well-being. Samantha, Mark, and numerous others inspire hope and share practical insights into living with lupus.

Conclusion: Adopting A Healthy Lifestyle

As we near the end of our trip through "Lupus Diet Solutions," it is important to reflect on the transformative potential of adopting a healthy lifestyle. Managing lupus is obviously difficult, but it can also be a liberating journey full with options that encourage healing and wellbeing. The insights offered in this book not only provide assistance, but also act as a reminder that you are in control of your health.

Embracing a Healthy Lifestyle

Living with lupus necessitates a comprehensive strategy that includes diet, lifestyle, and emotional health. The dietary ideas presented in this book—focusing on anti-inflammatory foods and limiting triggers—are essential for nurturing your body and alleviating symptoms. However, choosing a healthy lifestyle covers all aspects of your everyday life, not simply what you eat.

1. A commitment to Whole Foods:

Choosing organic, unprocessed foods indicates a commitment to supporting your body. Each meal provides an opportunity to refuel with vitamins, minerals, and antioxidants that boost your immune system and fight inflammation. This shift toward whole foods not only benefits your physical health, but it also fosters a greater appreciation for the products you eat.

2. Mindfulness Eating Practices:

A mindful approach to eating urges you to heed to your body's instincts. Paying attention to how different foods make you feel can help you figure out what works for you and what doesn't.

Mindfulness in eating can also make meals a relaxing, delightful event rather than a frantic necessity.

3. Lifestyle adjustments:

A healthy lifestyle requires physical activity, stress management, and a focus on sleep. Regular exercise—whether easy yoga, walking, or any other activity you enjoy—can improve mood, increase energy, and support general health. Furthermore, stress-reduction strategies like meditation, deep breathing, and simply spending time in nature might help you achieve a more balanced mental state.

4. Support systems:

Surrounding yourself with a supportive network is essential. Having friends, relatives, or support groups who understand your experience can make a big impact. Sharing experiences, problems, and achievements develops a feeling of community and gives the motivation you need to stick to your health goals.

5. Continuous Learning:

The journey to manage lupus is ongoing. Staying informed about new research, therapies, and dietary strategies empowers you. This book is simply one of many resources. Regularly seeking out new information allows you to adjust your techniques as needed, ensuring that your approach to health is dynamic and adaptable.

Encouragement for your journey ahead

Remember that every step of this trip is important. It is not about perfection, but about growth. Celebrate minor triumphs, such as trying a new recipe, feeling more energy, or just getting through a difficult day. Each positive improvement enhances your general health and well-being.

It's also critical to be kind towards yourself. Lupus treatment can be unexpected, with both good and poor days. Allow yourself the grace to handle these changes without judgement. Recognize your efforts and do not hesitate to seek assistance when necessary.

Connecting to the Community:

The lupus community is large and full of people who understand what you are going through. Engage with others via internet forums, local support groups, or social media. Sharing your story and learning from others can offer both comfort and useful advice for living with lupus.

Setting realistic goals:

Goal setting can be an effective motivator. Begin with attainable goals that are compatible with your lifestyle modifications. Whether it's committing to meal prep once a week, including more fruits and veggies into your meals, or starting a new fitness regimen, each modest goal lays the path for greater success.

Visualize Your Success:

Visualization is a great technique for changing your thinking. Take some time to imagine your ideal healthy lifestyle—how you feel, the activities you enjoy, and the vivacious energy you emit. This mental image might act as a guiding light, encouraging you to keep on your course.

Seek professional guidance:

Do not hesitate to seek the assistance of healthcare specialists such as certified dietitians, nutritionists, and therapists. Their knowledge can give specialized tactics that address your specific requirements, making your journey as effective and supportive as possible.

The Power of Perseverance

As you look ahead, recall the stories of those who came before you. Their experiences demonstrate the durability of the human spirit. Although managing lupus presents problems, it also provides chances for development, healing, and transformation. You may confidently traverse this road by making informed decisions and adopting a health-conscious lifestyle.

In conclusion, may this book serve as a springboard for your road to a healthier, more satisfying life. Lupus does not define you; rather, it is one of many aspects of your life. Accept the possibility of recovery and recognize that with each step you take, you are actively engaging in your own well-being. May your journey be full of hope, strength, and the delight of finding what it is to thrive.

<u>**Angela. O.**</u>

The end

101

www.ingramcontent.com/pod-product-compliance
Lightning Source LLC
Chambersburg PA
CBHW061246250726
48653CB00002B/528